Table o

Dedication

This book is dedicated to everyone at work. I feel you. I've had jobs where I sat all day, jobs where I stood all day, and jobs where I carried heavy awkward stuff. I've had horrible bosses that drove me to therapy and have run my own business where you lie awake at night wondering if you are going to make rent. I've scrounged for change in my car for gas money and borrowed $5.00 from friends so I could eat dinner. I've faced medical challenges and watched my mother die from cancer while my dad ran his own business and tried to figure out how to manage a teenage me.

I'm Type A and I'm a very hard worker. I take all of my jobs seriously and I've run myself into the ground doing it, sacrificing sleep, nutrition, my body, and my mind to succeed. I learned some things along the way. And I wrote this book with you in mind. Because I want you to be successful, abundant, prosperous...and alive to enjoy it all; to have a long, healthy, and full existence. So, for all of you, the head execs and the worker bees, I wrote this book. Enjoy!

And special thanks to my husband Michael for allowing my only-child, Capricorn, Type A, control-freak, driven self to thrive.

Kathy Gruver, PhD
Santa Barbara, CA

Also, a reminder that I am **NOT** a medical doctor and this book is not meant to take the place of your health care provider. I am not intending to diagnose or treat any illness.

Why I Wrote this Book

My first job ("job") was cleaning paint cans in my dad's paint store in Pittsburgh. I don't know that I did a particularly good job, but I loved spending the day with my dad, seeing him interact with all the customers, and I was learning about work. He taught me how to work the cash register and count change (the machine didn't do that for you). I helped with inventory and adding large columns of numbers. They were skills. Skills that set me up for later in life.

Then I did the requisite babysitting and my stint as a shift supervisor at Domino's Pizza, a little bit of waiting tables, and even worked as a house cleaner. When I launched out on my own, I landed in California, waiting tables at IHOP. Not, by any means, my dream job. But I did soon find myself in an office environment, with a briefcase and suit. I remember when a co-worker asked me to fax something and I approached the machine and realized I had no bloody idea how to work it. I felt stupid. I was embarrassed. She noticed and covertly showed me how. I should have just asked. I went from office job to office job, in between acting gigs. Now, I'm a fulltime massage therapist/hypnotherapist/author/speaker.

I share all this to let you know that I've had jobs of all kinds, jobs in corporate environments where stress was high and lax jobs where half the staff was high. I've had to quit and I've been laid off. I've had conflict with colleagues, bosses, bosses' wives, and been "written up" for discipline issues.

Work is hard. Even if you love what you do, there are challenges and days we just don't want to be there. I feel you. And this collection of information will help you to be healthier at your place of work, whether the office or the construction site. This is the companion piece to *Conquer Your Stress at Work*, so I'm not addressing any stress issues here, but everything on that subject is laid out in the other book. This is everything else I know, what I've learned about being healthy at work, whether you're sitting at a desk, standing at a bar, driving all day, or lifting heavy crap. Please enjoy these tips and let me know how I can help you be healthier at work. Find me at www.KathyGruver.com

Introduction to Office Health

More and more companies are talking about corporate wellness. But what exactly does that mean and how can it help your business? With the high cost of health care, the ramifications of injured employees, and the risk of Worker's Compensation claims, many corporations are instituting policies to encourage better health. Whether it's chair massage, gym memberships, yoga, stretching, or ergonomic consultations, companies are becoming proactive in keeping their staff healthy and well.

According to the National Institute of Occupational Safety and Health, repetitive stress injuries affect about 1.8 million workers per year. So, it is in the best interest of the company to keep everyone safe.

Carpal tunnel and tendinitis can be avoided with proper posture, stretching, breaks, nutrition, and station set-up. We can't just blame ergonomics for these problems, though. Forty years ago, secretaries didn't have the latest contoured chair or a consultant measuring how far their typewriter was from their eyes. They varied their activities, and even if their day was composed of just typing, they had to wind the tape, roll the paper, make corrections, etc. Now, with the word processor, we can type for hours, never having to change positions or move at all. We have convenienced ourselves into a state of injury. And the smaller the gadgets get, the harder it is on our arms and eyes. BlackBerry® devices, iPhones, and PDAs are contributing to finger and wrist issues. I know we need to use them, but counter that activity by putting them down occasionally and stretching.

We cannot hold technology solely responsible for these problems either; employees have to be conscious about their bodies and their health. Many staff work too long in one position without stopping. By law, breaks are provided, but I know many who don't take them. In many cases, there are imposed deadlines, too little staff, and too much work. We have to find the balance between productivity and our own wellbeing.

It is also common to find people eating poor quality food at their desks or never taking a break to walk around or go to the bathroom, let alone stretch and exercise. It is important that we listen to our bodies' cues and stop when we need to—every 50 minutes or so is ideal. It benefits everyone in the long run to take time to stretch, eat a nutritious meal or snack, and walk around in the sun for just five minutes.

And once the workday is over, it is important to stay active and fit. Working on the computer all day and then going home to play computer games is problematic from a health perspective. Management can't control what staff does outside the office, but logic dictates that this isn't the best choice. Try to find hobbies that use different parts than those you are already overusing at work. Data entry people who go home and knit, garden, and do beading are just asking for hand issues. And often times, it becomes a Worker's Comp problem. It is time for us all to take responsibility for ourselves and our wellness. Stretch, eat right, and exercise. I will teach you how to do all these things and more.

As a boss, letting your staff know that you care about their wellbeing and health is a way to ensure better productivity and loyalty. We will look at ways to encourage better office health, and I will give you tips and hints to fit in fitness, revamp your kitchen to provide healthier foods, and stretches and exercises that can be easily incorporated into your day. Let's get underway!

Office Wellness During Cold and Flu Season

When cold and flu season is upon us, expect sneezes, sniffling, and snot from the coworker who just borrowed your stapler. In an ideal world, people would not show up to work sick. But with the economy the way it is and people apprehensive about missing work for fear of losing a paycheck or losing their job, we must take the initiative to protect our own health. Here are some tips to keep you healthy in the workplace.

Hygiene

Let's start with the basics. Our mothers were right: hand washing can protect you from germs. Make sure you wash your hands with soap and hot water and get between your fingers and under your fingernails. I know a lot of office staff that keep hand sanitizer at their desks and disinfectant wipes close by in case they are covering someone else's phone or using their supplies. In between hand washing, avoid touching your face and eyes too. Don't become too germ-phobic though, as being around germs can actually help you build up your immune system.

Supplements

Taking a multivitamin containing extra vitamin C and zinc has been shown to help prevent colds and speed recovery time. Some people mega dose on vitamin C, but we can only absorb a certain amount at a time (opinions vary on how much), so if you are going to take extra vitamin C, spread out the dose. An excess of vitamin C can cause loose bowel movements and gas, which is a good hint that you've had too much. I personally am a big fan of Airborne™. Airborne™ was developed by a teacher and contains 17 vitamins, minerals, and herbs. I find it works for me and could work well for you too.

Herbs like Echinacea and Golden Seal have properties that can help speed healing of colds and flu. Garlic is another helpful herb and can be taken in your food or bought in a "de-odorized" supplement form like Kyolic™. There are numerous supplement formulas on the market to boost your immune system; I recommend trying some and seeing what you like best.

One of my favorites is Wellness Formula. When I was working long hours on the film set, many producers made it a requirement that we all take it to stay healthy.

Homeopathy

Homeopathic remedies are a safe and easy way to try to stave off illness. Homeopathy works on the principle of "like cures like," and the remedy is determined by examining a combination of very specific symptoms like: Is your entire nose stuffy or just the right side? Does your headache get better when you drink cold water? Are you craving salt? Is your face flushed? Are you cranky and do you want to be left alone? Answering a series of questions such as these can guide you to the right single remedy.

Combination remedies are also readily available and tend to mingle the most common remedies for the ailment. There are remedies simply named Cold and Flu, and there is an effective combination called Oscillococcinum™, which has worked for me in the past. You can enquire at your favorite health food store or contact a trained professional.

Think Yourself Well

We have enormous power in our minds. Studies show that we can actually boost our immune system by visualizations and affirmations. If you are afraid of every germ and sure that so and so from your office is infecting you, chances are you are going to catch something. Our attitude and what we say in our minds strongly affects what happens in our bodies. Repeating to yourself that you are healthy and well or that your immune system is strong can actually prevent you from catching the latest thing.

De-Stress Yourself!

So much research has been done on the effects of stress on the immune system. And let's be clear, it's not so much the stress, it's your reaction to the stress. If you can take things in stride and make sure you allow yourself some downtime to process all of what is happening in your life, you can keep that immune system healthier. And if you are paranoid about getting sick, you are adding stress, which is decreasing the effectiveness of the immune system, which will be more apt to let an illness take hold. For my five-point de-stress program, pick up *Conquer Your Stress at Work*.

Keep Drinking Water

Not only should we have a large amount of water for health in general, but it is even more important when we are sick. Water can help thin out mucous and keep our noses and lungs clear. Tea, broth, and juice are good too; just make sure you are not adding artificial sweeteners or getting juice that is filled with high-fructose corn syrup.

Try to Be As Happy As You Can

I have watched people who are always sick. You know them; they catch everything that comes around. And they always try to blame someone for "getting them sick." I have noticed that, more often than not, these people are basically unhappy. Perhaps they don't like their jobs; maybe their marriage is less than ideal, or they could be experiencing some level of depression. Whatever the source of the unhappiness, I think that if they could be happier, they would also be healthier. Illness is very often used as an excuse to not face something. I would suggest to someone that is always sick that they examine what else is going on in their lives. It is sometimes a really hard question to ask ourselves, but worth the work if we desire to stay healthy and have a long and productive life.

Western Medicine

What about western medicine? What does it have to offer at this time of year? Not much, frankly. Some people rush to get their flu shots. These are recommended for older adults, children, and people with compromised immune systems. Every year the formula changes in an effort to battle the virus of the year. Some people have found that the flu shot makes them sick, and others get the flu anyway. I have read numerous reports that the flu shot increases the risk for Alzheimer's disease from the additives like mercury and aluminum contained in the vaccine.

I have also seen evidence that the vaccine doesn't do anything at all. Remember that the flu shot is a combination of many chemical and natural compounds, some of which can have side effects. I am not recommending against the flu shot, but rather encouraging you to be informed before you make any medical or natural health choice.

Antibiotics are not going to help you get rid of a cold either. A cold is caused by a virus, and antibiotics work on bacteria. However, if a cold develops into an upper respiratory infection or sinus infection, antibiotics may be appropriate. Some doctors recommend flu anti-virals, which are effective if taken at the first signs of being sick (within the first two days). It can decrease the length of the flu by one or two days and makes you less contagious to others, according to the CDC website. These specific drugs will not work on a cold, just the flu.

And remember, the sneezing, runny nose, and coughing that come with a cold is the body's effort to get the bad stuff out. If you go overboard in repressing the symptoms with drugs, you may prolong the illness. One of your best defenses is rest, so try to get plenty of it and take the time off work if possible!

The Office Environment:
Healthy Additions to Your Office

For those of us that spend hours on end at the office, it's great to have some resources there that we can use to be healthier. Here are a few suggestions.

First Aid

Most offices keep a medicine chest in the office. As well as pain reducers and cold medicine, keep some multivitamins and minerals on hand. I also recommend some immune boosters like Wellness Formula™ or Airborne™. If you provide your employees with what is needed to keep them illness free, you'll have healthier and more motivated employees.

Get Moving

Many companies offer a gym membership or have a gym on the premises. If you can't go that route, at least provide a few hand weights, a yoga ball, or exercise bands. These are small additions that will help your staff fit in fitness during their busy day. And since we all have to leave our desks at some point, keep some charts of stretches and easy exercises (like those given later in this book) in the break room or kitchen. When people head for a snack or to the bathroom, it's the perfect time to take a break to stretch and move their body. You can also post the stretch of the week near the copy or fax machine and encourage people to stretch while they're waiting.

Have scheduled breaks throughout the day, when everyone in the office stops and stretches or exercises. If you have every one participating, even for a few minutes a day, you'll have a built-in buddy system. If you want to take that concept further, sponsor an office Olympics or Biggest Loser contest. Get everyone involved and supporting each other. Start a point system for exercise or weight loss. Put a big chart on the wall and give everyone stars for their achievements like we had in grade school.

Back to the Kitchen

Have options for things other than soda, cookies, processed foods, and artificial sweeteners. Stevia is a great option instead of Equal® or Splenda®. Many people have reactions to those chemical sweeteners, and eliminating them from the office might also eliminate issues that people didn't even connect to the artificial sweetener, like headaches, anxiety, and feelings of hyperactivity.

MSG is another problem-causing substance that is commonly found in processed foods and chips. Have whoever does your purchasing avoid buying these products. Again, many people have reactions like headaches, anxiety, nausea, hyperactivity, and intestinal issues from MSG.

I also recommend eliminating soda. Diet or regular soda has no nutritional value, keeps people from drinking other healthy beverages like water, and can lead to health problems. High-fructose corn syrup, which sweetens most mainstream sodas, has been linked to obesity and type-2 diabetes. The diet variety contains artificial sweeteners which, as well as the above-mentioned problems, also suppress the production of leptin, a chemical in the brain that tells us when we're full. So, we wind up eating more. Not much of a diet plan.

The Office Environment

Let the sun shine in. Try to get as much natural light in your office as you can. This can be difficult in a space with many cubicles and moveable walls. If you own the building, Solartubes and skylights might be an option. You can also replace your florescent lights with full spectrum light bulbs. These seem to cause less eyestrain and prevent people from getting Seasonal Affective Disorder (SAD) during the winter months.

Bring nature inside. Plants can not only brighten a room but also provide oxygen and clean the air. Here are a few that are especially known for their oxygenation power:

- Reed palm
- Dwarf date palm
- Boston fern
- English ivy

- Peace lily
- Australian sword fern
- Rubber plant
- Weeping fig

I see many offices with artificial plants; I really recommend getting live plants instead. There are services that will bring plants and flowers into your office and maintain them for you. One of the downsides of artificial plants is that they tend to collect dust and other particles, which might irritate allergen-sensitive people. Turn to real nature if you can.

And speaking of sensitive people, we are seeing more and more folks developing multiple chemical sensitivities. The office is an environment ripe with these compounds. Toner fluid, copy-machine chemicals, out-gassing from carpet and assembled furniture, even the smell from markers, whiteout, and pens can put someone over the edge of having physical reactions. So much of that is out of our control, but try to make the best choices when looking at office chairs, carpet, and paint.

Speaking of chairs, provide your staff with what they need to be healthy at their desks. Listen to their concerns about chair height, computer placement, and office setup. And make sure the chairs are good quality and fit the employees. I had a client that had to wait 6 months to get her chair approved because "only the management was allowed to have chairs with arms." I was appalled by that and disappointed that she ended up injured because of such a ridiculous and outdated policy.

An Example of What You Can Do in Your Personal Space
I had a client who was incredibly stressed out. She was a financial advisor and managed people's millions. She was working 10 or 12-hour days, not leaving her desk, not eating lunch, and generally going crazy. She was not productive, not sleeping, and stressed beyond belief. She came to me for a stress management session. I asked her when her last vacation was, and it had been three or four years ago. I asked her where her favorite vacation spot was, and she said it was Hawaii; sitting on the beach was her perfect escape.

She had the advantage of having her own office space with a door. I asked her if she was allowed to do whatever she wanted to do with that space, and she answered in the affirmative. I told her to go ahead and paint the walls, make them a nice sea blue or something that reminded her of the sky. I advised her to put a photo on her desk of herself at the beach, or better yet, her legs looking out towards the ocean as if she were sitting in a chaise lounge. I also had her buy a scented candle that smelled like the ocean or coconut, whatever got her in that relaxing place. She also bought a sound machine that had the sound of the ocean. I asked her if she had a computer; she answered that she had two. I asked her what her backdrop was on the computer; she said that swirly thing that came with the computer. I told her to get rid of the swirly thing and get scenes of the ocean or the beach or palm trees. And the final piece, and this was many years ago, I asked her if she had one of those big old desks with the drawer to the right for files that is now filled with crap. She said she did. I asked her what was in that drawer. She answered, "Crap." I told her to take the crap out and put in a bucket filled with sand. So, whenever she needed to, she could turn on the sound machine, light the candle, stare at the picture frame or the computer and put her hand in the bucket of sand. We managed to bring Hawaii to her. And, because the brain thinks what we are fantasizing about is real, it took her on a vacation in her office.

Even if you don't have your own office space or if you're in a job that's in a van, bar, hair salon, or car, you have the ability to have something as a reminder that takes you to your relaxing space. Perhaps it's something in your car so that as you drive to and from work, you can take an extra minute to relax either before or after your shift. Maybe you have something in your purse or an app on your phone that is a reminder, a trigger that it's time to relax. Something on your key ring or in your truck. The list of possibilities is endless, if you think about it. We are living in a time where stress is higher than ever, and if we can take those moments of what we need to remind us to go to our special place, we are going to have an advantage.

Nutrition at Work:
Feed me.

Healthy Treats at the Office

I remember working in offices and getting so excited that it was Wednesday. Why? Because Wednesday was Donut Day!!!!! Or Bagel Thursday or Pizza Party Friday. I loved it. It saved me money and it was food I didn't normally get to have. What a treat. And I remember women moaning about the food, sneaking guiltily in to the kitchen and grabbing their 5th donut, mumbling something about their butt. Why do we do this to ourselves? 1. Have some self-control. 2. When you do snack, don't feel bad about allowing yourself to have something that you want. Don't have five and feel bad, have one and eat it with joy! You don't need to explain yourself, or apologize. See, this is where I don't like "diets". Because diets tell you you have do this thing 100% and if you "cheat," you fail.

I believe in the 80/20 rule. 80% of the time do the best you can. 20%, you have a treat (a treat, not a cheat). So eat the donut and do it with consciousness and grace.
Or, better yet...let's have healthy things at the office. I do massage at a company that has fresh produce delivered every week, so there is always something amazing to snack on. When you surround the staff with healthy options, they are going to take advantage of them.

To help your eating habits at the office be healthy, make sure what you've eaten <u>away</u> from the office will sustain you. Try to make time for a hearty breakfast before you get in your car to zoom off for the day. Many people skip this essential meal, but it is important for energy, thought processes, and weight maintenance. I suggest a morning meal that has a combination of protein, fats, and carbohydrates. This gives you the best variety of nutrients and long and short-term energy supplies. A breakfast of eggs, meat, fish, nuts, etc. is a great start to the morning. And remember, you don't have to have "breakfast food" for breakfast. I often have left over dinner for breakfast. There's no reason you can't have steak, chicken, salad, or fish for breakfast.

I don't have to tell you how important it is to drink pure water throughout the day. Most offices have a water cooler or bottled water available. Some also provide coffee, tea, juice, and soda. I'm not opposed to coffee or tea; however, relying on caffeine to get you through the day may backfire when the afternoon crash occurs. Caffeine late in the day can cause evening wakefulness and anxiety, so don't depend on artificial stimulants. And if you are adding artificial sweetener to your coffee or tea, it might be causing health issues.

Juice is a great beverage, but make sure it's not just colored, sweetened water with some juice flavor added. Unfortunately, pure juice is rather expensive, and most of what you get in the store has very little fruit in it. Read the labels.

As you know by now, I'm not a fan of soda. Diet or regular, soda has no nutritional value, and its consumption can lead to poor health. As I've said before (and will probably mention again), high-fructose corn syrup has not only been linked to obesity, but may also be contributing to the rise in cases of diabetes and hyperactivity. Soda is high in phosphorus, which leeches calcium and other minerals from our bodies. And artificial sweetener contained in the diet variety is a dangerous chemical. Numerous illnesses have been associated with these compounds including headaches and migraines, anxiety attacks, MS, and seizures, and it has been shown to decrease leptin production in the brain, which tells us when we are full. If you are a sodaholic, please consider switching to a healthier habit. And if you need to sweeten your coffee or tea, try a natural product like honey, sugar, xylitol, or stevia (my favorite).

There are always one or two staffers that practically live in the kitchen. They're always there, grabbing a handful of this or another piece of that. If this is you, why are you in there? Heading to the kitchen is a great distraction from our work, which can be both good and bad. I do encourage taking breaks, but munching through them is not the healthiest choice. If you find yourself wandering to the food area, ask if you are really hungry, or if you are bored, anxious, angry, or just looking for a diversion. Many people struggling with weight realize that they eat to satisfy some other aspect that is currently unfulfilled. Emotional eating can lead to weight and health issues. If you aren't hungry, explore why you might be in the kitchen and what issues might need to be addressed.

If you are hungry and need a snack, select fruit, nuts, or popcorn as opposed to processed foods, cookies, or chips. Many conventional snack foods like Doritos® contain MSG, which is an excitotoxin and causes a negative reaction in sensitive people. Unfortunately, MSG is often hidden in the ingredients as something else, like "spices" or "natural flavors". If you are sensitive to MSG, make sure you avoid those hidden sources.

As I mentioned before, it's very important to take breaks throughout the day. And lunchtime is no exception. I understand, there are days when there is a deadline or something just can't wait, but making a habit of working through lunch and eating at your desk is an unhealthy practice. Our digestive system works best in a relaxed environment, so shoving food in your mouth as you're coding and stressing about a deadline is going to lead to stomach and bowel issues. If you're rushing through lunch, you're also not chewing enough, which is harder on the stomach. Take some time, relax for a few minutes, chew, and enjoy your food. And, make sure what you're eating is real food and not a processed "frankenfood". It is much more convenient to choose a pre-packaged microwavable meal, but the nutrition is often not present. And many of these foods contain trans fats, MSG, high-fructose corn syrup, additives, preservatives, or ingredients that have been genetically modified. We are not only getting subpar nutrition from these foods, but the added components may be making us sick, fat, and tired. Pack lunch from your home or eat at a healthier restaurant in town.

We can see that better nutrition helps us to be more present, productive and healthy. Try changing your office eating habits. You'll feel better, and your body AND your boss will thank you.

Add and Subtract from Your Diet at Work:
More Details about How to Eat Better

As quickly as you change the channel on the TV, the concept of what is good and bad for you changes as well. Remember when we were told that butter was bad and we should all eat margarine? Eeek. Or that eggs were an evil food? Unfortunately, a lot of our food information comes to us from who has the money for the advertising and what lobbyist got their wish that week in Washington. Here's my take on the things to add and subtract for better health.

Add a high-quality multivitamin and mineral supplement. If you can find these from whole food sources, all the better. We need <u>minerals</u> for all functions of the body, so don't forget them either. Everyone hears so much about calcium, but remember, there are so many more that are needed, like copper, zinc, manganese, and molybdenum. And calcium needs other minerals like magnesium to assimilate it. Magnesium, which is depleted in our bodies during times of stress, is also is great for fixing constipation, muscle aches, mood and sleep issues, and PMS.

Eliminate soda, regular AND diet. Regular soda contains high-fructose corn syrup, which has been linked to obesity in some studies, and diet drinks contains dangerous artificial sweeteners. Both contain artificial colors, phosphorus (which depletes minerals from the body), and carbonation (which can be hard on the system). And soda keeps you from drinking other healthy beverages.

Add amino acids. This is a commonly overlooked addition, but amino acids are the building blocks of protein that we need for our bodies to function properly. Many are "essential," meaning the body can't manufacture them and often we don't get enough in our food, especially vegetarians. I recommend L-Tryptophan for people experiencing sleep or mood disorders, but don't take this if you're on SSRIs (Selective Serotonin Reuptake Inhibitors) for depression.

Eliminate milk, unless you're a baby, a baby cow, or drinking raw, unpasteurized, un-homogenized milk straight from an organic cow in a wild field. A few milk facts: we are the only species that drinks other species' milks, we are the only species that drinks milk after we are weaned at about the age of two, and genetically, most of us lose the ability to digest milk as adults. Many people are lactose sensitive and cannot handle milk products. I see many parents complaining of their children getting repeated ear infections and having to take lots of antibiotics. Often the child is allergic to milk and it's manifesting as ear problems. I recommend they take their kids off milk to see if the condition clears, but many are reluctant. rBGH is a dangerous hormone, and most conventional cows are filled with antibiotics. Also, in order to produce milk, the cows are basically tricked in to being constantly pregnant, so those hormones (and antibiotics) are getting in to us. There are many other ways to get the needed vitamins and minerals.

Add essential fatty acids, specifically omega-3s. It used to be that we obtained omega-3 and -6 in equal quantities, but because of our change in diet (more meats, corn, and soy oil), we are now getting far more omega-6, which might be contributing to the rise in depression and inflammation. Add flax seed or fish oil. It's good for the skin, mood, and heart.

Eliminate artificial sweetener, which has been around a long time, with Sweet 'N Low® (Saccharin) being the first used back in the '70s. Saccharin has been linked to bladder cancer, breathing problems, headaches, skin eruptions, diarrhea, and larger reactions in people allergic to Sulfa drugs. If you really, really MUST have artificial sweeteners, this one seems to be the most benign, and since it's been around the longest, it has the most research behind it.

NutraSweet™, Equal®, Sugar Twin® (Aspartame) are a big no-no to me. Aspartame has been linked to cancer, hair loss, depression, dementia, headaches, dizziness, nausea, vomiting, fatigue, seizures, and increased hunger!!! Studies show it may reduce the production/reception of hormone leptin (which tells us when we're full) in the brain, thus we eat more. There have not been intensive studies on this chemical, and many scientists feel that the FDA never should have approved it. Once in the body, it converts to methyl alcohol, which then converts to formaldehyde (you know, that thing they embalm dead bodies with). In 1988, 80% of the complaints to the FDA were about aspartame, yet it remains on the market and is found in countless products. Read the labels carefully!

Splenda® (Sucralose), which is the newest addition to the sweetener family, contains chlorine and has been shown to cause gastrointestinal issues, wheezing, coughing, depression, mood swings, and its effects on animals have only been studied in the short-term. I had a client that was having chest pains and breathing issues. Upon examination of what might be different in his life, he had recently switched to Splenda® from Equal®. When he eliminated the substance, his chest and breathing issues went away (as did his ER visits). These substances act as excitotoxins in the brain...and we wonder why we have so much ADHD...

Add probiotics, which are the good bugs that live in our intestines. Yogurt is great, but not enough. If you've ever been on antibiotics, these are essential. Make sure you get one with 60 billion CFUs (colony forming units). This good bacterium not only keeps your digestive system healthy, but they also produce needed vitamins.

Eliminate trans fats, and anything with hydrogenised or partially-hydrogenated oils. Even if it says No Trans Fats, if it has anything hydrogenated in it, it contains trans fats. These contribute to inflammation in the body and can lead to cancer and heart disease. Skip the margarine and use real butter. And it's believed that trans fats stay in the system for 6 months.

Add digestive enzymes. Many of us have compromised digestive systems, and as we age, its function often declines. We need enzymes for every function in the body. Protease, lipase, and amylase are the most common. Bromelain and papain, which come from papaya and pineapple, might help with arthritis pain and inflammation in the body.

Eliminate high-fructose corn syrup. Please don't believe the propaganda TV commercials. Corn is natural, but HFCS isn't, as far as I'm concerned, even if they do change the name to "corn sugar". It could be making this country obese and diabetic. There is evidence that fructose suppresses leptin, the hormone that gives the sensation of fullness, and causes a raise in triglycerides and insulin resistance. Make up your own mind; the rate of obesity almost identically mirrors the rate of our HFCS consumption. See the chart below:

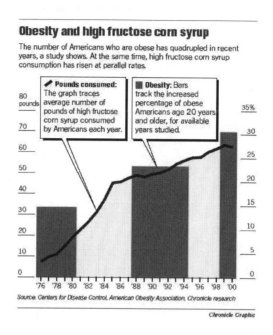

Obesity and high fructose corn syrup

The number of Americans who are obese has quadrupled in recent years, a study shows. At the same time, high fructose corn syrup consumption has risen at parallel rates.

✎ **Pounds consumed:** The graph traces average number of pounds of high fructose corn syrup consumed by Americans each year.

▉ **Obesity:** Bars track the increased percentage of obese Americans age 20 years and older, for available years studied.

Source: Centers for Disease Control, American Obesity Association, Chronicle research

Chronicle Graphic

And let's just say the research is correct and HFCS is just as safe as sugar—it's still a highly processed food, which I recommend eliminating, and it's probably genetically modified, which I also think should be avoided (see below).

Add more fiber and water so you poop more. Yes, I'm about to talk about poop. Most Americans' bowel habits are less than optimal. Make sure you get enough water, exercise, and fiber. There are two types of fiber, soluble and insoluble. Get a good combination of both. Aim for 2-3 bowel movements a day (Yeah…a day) and note your transit time. Food should appear at the other end of you in 16-24 hours. You can check this with sunflower seeds (with the shells on), corn, or beets. If the time is too slow, you will be accumulating feces in the colon and absorbing toxins and if it's too fast, you'll be missing out on needed nutrients.

Eliminate genetically modified organisms (GMOs). The most commonly genetically modified substances are corn and soy. Not the corn that you eat at the BBQ and not the good soy products like edamame. The bad ones are mainly turned into high-fructose corn syrup and soy protein and soy oil. These products are in most processed foods and trying to eliminate them can be a challenge. Buy organic or products that are labeled NON-GMO. Learn about Monsanto, the company responsible for most of the GMOs. Two recommendations are *The World According to Monsanto* and *The Future of Food*, two great films on our food, GMOs, and farming.

Wonder what those little stickers on our produce mean? Here's a guide:

Conventional produce gets a four-digit number.
Organic produce gets a five-digit number that starts with 9.
Genetically modified items also get a five-digit code, but that code starts with 8.

Examples
4139: Conventional apple
94139: Organic apple
84139: GMO apple

Luckily, at this point there is very little, if any, produce that is a GMO except for some papayas from Hawaii and crookneck squash. Organic is still best, though, to avoid pesticides, fungicides, and chemical fertilizer.

The final elimination: MSG. This is a dangerous excitotoxin that causes hyperactivity, nausea, headaches, flushing, and racing heart in sensitive individuals. It can also cause swelling, diarrhea, vomiting, stiffness, achiness, mood issues, anxiety, panic attacks, migraines, insomnia, dizziness, asthma, rash, and many, many more symptoms. It does not have to be labeled as MSG, so you might be consuming it without your knowledge. It is known by many names and is common in processed foods. Here are just a few:

- Glutamate, Glutamic acid, Gelatin, Monosodium glutamate, Calcium caseinate, Textured protein, Monopotassium glutamate, Sodium caseinate, Yeast nutrient, Yeast extract, Yeast food, Autolyzed yeast,

Hydrolyzed protein (any protein that is hydrolyzed), Hydrolyzed corn gluten, Natrium glutamate (natrium is Latin/German for sodium), Flavorings, Seasonings.

I know this seems like a pretty intense list of things to get rid of and you wonder what is left to eat. What our grandparents ate...natural, unprocessed foods. Your body will thank you and you'll see your health improve!

Exercise:
Ways to Fit in Fitness

We all know we have to exercise for our bodies, but consider what it does for our minds. Exercise releases endorphins and other feel good hormones in the brain. It usually leads to better sleep. It is a moving meditation, especially something like running, swimming, or walking. And there is no reason you can't throw in positive talk while you're doing it. It gives us a better personal body image and often, when we start doing things that are healthy, other unhealthy things drop away as well. After running 10 miles and feeling great, we are less apt to want to pig out on chocolate cake. Exercise has been known to decrease depression also. Regular exercise also helps condition the immune system so we stay healthier. Many people daydream during exercise and find that, with their minds clearer, they can come up with solutions to problems and options for their issues. And exercise itself seems to act as a buffer against stress.

The most important thing about exercise is to find what works best for <u>you</u>! Some people run, swim, walk, golf, surf, or play soccer, volleyball, or badminton—the list is endless. I choose to dance. Dance not only strengthens my body, but it keeps my mind sharp and healthy. And it's good for my spirit. In fact, a recent study on life satisfaction showed that people who dance have more life satisfaction that people who do most other exercise.

To add in exercise, first off, pick something that you will enjoy. Start out slowly and be gentle with yourself. Get others to do it with you. Schedule it in so you know you have time for it. Change it up if you think you will get bored with one thing. And set realistic goals. You'll find as you reach them that you'll be even more inspired to continue.

Fitting in fitness at work can be a challenge, especially with shift work or if you are running your own business. A few tips:

- Try to do the opposite of what you do all day. So, if you are on your feet all day, do a non-standing exercise like bike riding or swimming. If you sit all day, move in a different way to work out.

- Keep dumbbells or bands at the office. There is no reason while you are on hold or listening in to a conference call that you can't do some exercise. I have a client that keeps weights next to the toilet and she does arm curls while she takes care of other business, the ultimate multitasking!
- Park further away and walk. Walk to the bathroom on a different floor or in a different part of the building. Go outside and around the building on the way to the bathroom.

Every little bit counts!

Stretches

I wanted to include some stretches because I think they are one of the most important parts of a workday. Ideally, do these twice a day and hold for 30 seconds on a side. Do not stretch through pain. If it hurts, stop. Thanks to my models Michael and Elaine.

These are perfect for arm, hand and wrist issues.

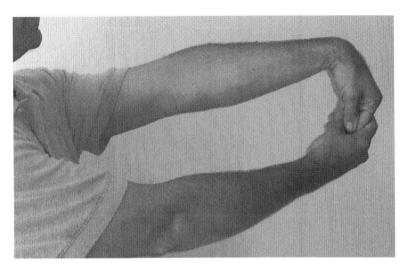

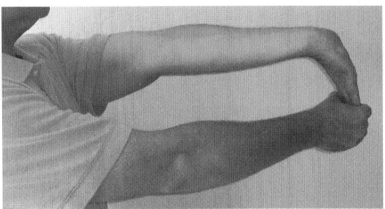

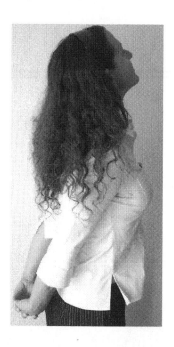

Especially if you are at a desk all day you want to keep your chest stretched out.

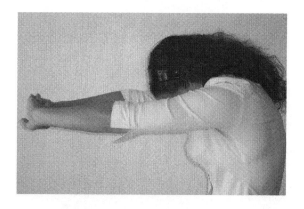

Great stretch for the upper back.

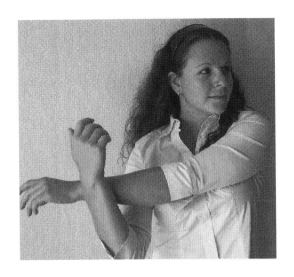

Ways to keep the shoulders stretched out.

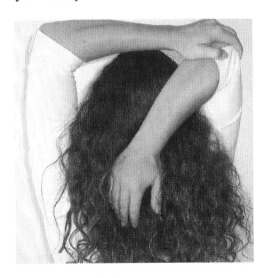

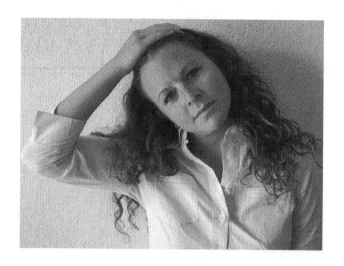

Keep your neck stretched. Just lay the hand across your head, don't pull. You can deepen this by anchoring the hanging hand (not pictured) on something or holding a weight.

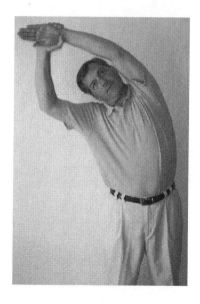

Don't forget the side of the body

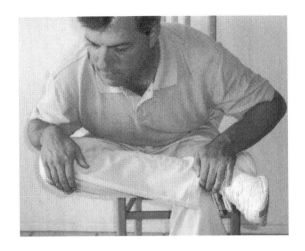

This is a great stretch for the piriformis, which is a common cause of sciatica and low back pain.

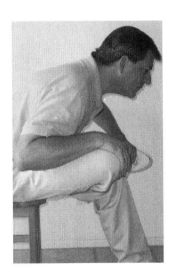

Another view of the piriformis stretch.

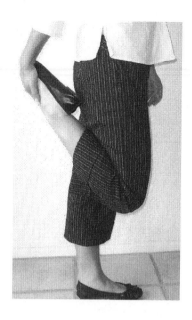

Stretch for the quads. Avoid this if you have bad knees.

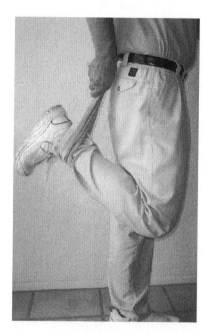

If you need some help you can use a towel or belt, seen above.

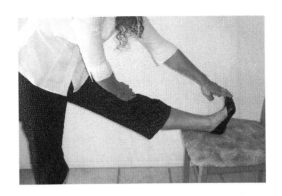

And those hamstrings!!

If You Sit All Day

-Make sure you change your position frequently.
-Get up and stretch at least once an hour.
-Make sure your chair and desk setup is appropriate for your size, shape, and tasks.

Don't sit like this!

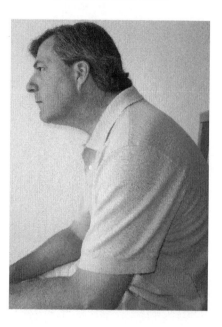

Very bad posture. This leads to shoulder, neck and upper back issues, and what is called sternum loading.

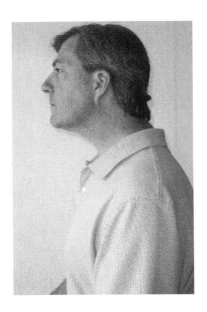

This is common posture for people with vision problems. This is also horrible for the neck.

Sit like this!

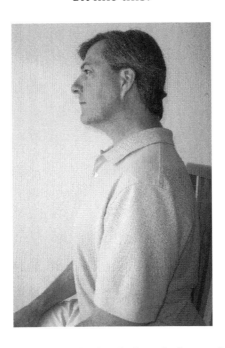

Much better, straight back, head above the neck.

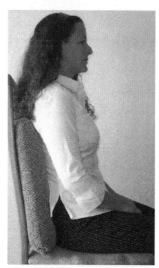

You can always use pillows and bolsters to enhance your posture.

-Try a standing desk for part of the day, or sitting on a yoga ball or a kneeling chair.
-Stretch at least once an hour (I repeated that on purpose and you may hear it again.)
-When off work, don't do exercises or activities that involve more sitting.
-Stay active.
-Walk around as much as you can during day.
-And hey, try stretching ;)

If You Sit All Day in the Car

-Get out of the car and stretch.
-Adjust your seat to a slightly different position occasionally.
-Take advantage of cruise control, if even for a few minutes at a time, to move that right leg around.
-Stretch your arms and neck if it's safe to do so.
-If you are tired, please rest. Pull over and close your eyes. Too many people power through and it ends disastrously.

If You Use Your Arms and Hands All Day

I'm not just talking about computer folks here, this applies to hairdressers, nail salon workers, massage therapists, assembly line workers, you name it:

-STRETCH THOSE ARMS!
-If possible with your job, change tasks so it's not totally the same movement all day.
-When you get home, don't do more stuff with your hands. Assembling small pieces all day and then going home and gardening and knitting isn't the best idea.
-Get bodywork on those arms. My husband uses a rolling pin on my forearms. It's heaven.
-Make sure the setup of your workstation is such that your posture stays healthy.
-Don't slouch or thrust your head forward (see examples in the "If You Sit All Day" chapter).

If You Are in Awkward Positions All Day

So, you spend your day under houses, under cars, laying flooring, etc.

-Please, please, please stretch.
-Get massage and chiropractic.
-Keep your nutrition as optimal as possible.
-Have a team of people that help keep you healthy.
-Do what it takes to keep your body strong and flexible. And if it hurts, stop! I know that's hard to when you need a paycheck or you are the job, but hurting yourself permanently isn't going to help you either. And this applies to all of us.

If You Stand All Day

-If you are having low back pain, check to see if you have a leg length difference and work with therapies to fix that.
-Sit, stretch, bend and lean when you can.
-Make sure you have fabulous footwear and consider insoles or orthotics to help take the pressure off.
-If you stand in the same place/position all day, try having a small box near your station that you can put one leg up on to take pressure off your feet and low back. And try to not to stand on the hard floor without some kind of padding or squishy mat beneath you.
-When off the job, don't do activities that involve more standing.

If You Lift Heavy ~~Shit~~ Stuff

This used to be one of the most common causes of Worker's Comp injuries, now it's been surpassed by repetitive stress injuries.

-Use your legs, engage your core.
-Make sure if something hurts, you take care of it.
-Use a brace if you need to, but over time, that can actually weaken your core and back.
-Do exercises on your time off to keep you healthy during your workday.
-Take some high-quality vitamin and mineral supplements and make sure you're eating enough protein to keep your body fueled.

Pain
Not tonight honey...

Headaches have been plaguing humans probably since humans have been in existence. And though they do offer a traditional excuse for avoiding intimacy, headaches can also interfere with daily functioning and take the joy out of life. This is an older statistic but still valid. According to the National Headache Association:

- 45% of respondents missed at least 5 family or social events in the last year because of a headache
- Nearly 30% have missed up to 5 days of work each month due to headache
- 25% of respondents reported that their coworkers resent the time they spend away from work due to a headache
- 20% of respondents reported their family and friends tend to resent them for missing events because of headaches

And an average of $1500/year is being spent on prescriptions, not to mention over-the-counter drugs like Advil® and Excedrin® Migraine.

Here are some causes and solutions for that pain in the head that you might not have thought of. The first thing I'd ask you to explore are side-effects from prescription drugs. Often, headaches can be caused by something you are already taking. Even if you've been on the drug for a while, side-effects can still develop. I was prone to horrible migraines and was tested for every disease under the sun. I was also put on numerous migraine medications, including Imitrex. Years later, when I decided to be drug-free, I got off the birth control pill. Miraculously, my headaches completely disappeared. Doing some research, I found that headaches are a common side effect of oral contraceptives. I could have saved myself years of pain and extra medication had someone just read the Prescription Drug Reference Guide. Look at your prescriptions and check for common side effects to see if they might be to blame. WebMD (www.webmd.com) is a great resource, as is the PDR

(Prescription Drug Reference). Also, a lot of headache medications can cause what are called "rebound headaches," which means that over time you must take more and more of the drug to get it to work. You might decide to talk to your doctor about trying a different prescription or getting off them all together. Of course, never stop taking a prescription without discussing this with your doctor first, as many prescriptions need to be gotten off of slowly.

Another common culprit for headaches is food sensitivities. With so many additives, flavorings, artificial colors and sweeteners, and MSG being added to our food, it's no wonder that people are having more headaches. You can take a food sensitivity test like the LEAP test (which differs from traditional allergy testing that your MD would do) to see if you are vulnerable to certain foods. You could also try keeping a food diary. Chart your daily intake of all foods and drinks and when your headaches occur. Over time, you might be able to see a pattern develop that will lead you to eliminate certain foods. Whether you decide to keep a food diary or not, there are common triggers that could be avoided as an experiment. Many people are sensitive to aged cheeses, chocolate, beer, and red wine. Try getting these out of your diet for at least six weeks to see if there is improvement in your symptoms. MSG is a repeat offender for headaches and migraines, as are artificial sweeteners like aspartame and sucralose. MSG doesn't have to be labeled in most food, and you can see some of the aliases for MSG in my nutrition section. These are huge instigators when it comes to headaches.

In the food diary, it would also be helpful to note stress level, menstrual phase, and level of physical activity. Stress is definitely a contributing factor to headaches. We tend to boost our shoulders up to our ears during stressful times, and that muscle tension can lead to headaches. Clenching our jaw also adds to the problem. Many people not only grind during the night but also clamp their jaws shut during their workday. My observation is, if you wake up with a headache, nine times out of ten, you were clenching and should work on relaxing your jaw. A mouth guard can help, but often people continue to grind and chew right though them. Also avoid gum-chewing and eating chewing-intensive foods like jerky if you are prone to jaw tension.

Hormonal changes can also lead to headaches. Many women experience headaches as part of their premenstrual symptoms or suddenly get them as they experience menopause. Making sure you get plenty of rest during this time is key, as is reducing your stress and eating right. See if your headaches at this time of month might be telling you to slow down and look inward to see if you are taking good enough care of yourself. Sometimes, our bodies are trying to communicate something to us through pain.

Sometimes our bodies get out of alignment, the same way our cars do. If the cervical (neck) vertebrae go "out," we might experience headaches. A chiropractor can offer help in this arena, as can an osteopath. Multiple visits might be necessary, but relief can usually be found. And keep an eye on your posture. I had a client having horrible headaches and neck pain. We finally figured out that she was craning the phone between her neck and shoulder and it was causing horrible issues.

Consider having your eyes checked. A computer screen that is too close or too far away or an outdated prescription for your glasses can definitely contribute to headaches. I've personally found that staring at small devices like my cell phone causes eyestrain, leading to a headache. Try to work on your full-size computer when you can.

We know that drinking too much alcohol can cause that next-day symptom of a headache. Even if you think you didn't drink enough to be hung over, think about the circumstances surrounding your consumption. Did you have enough food in your body? Were you staying hydrated? What was the alcohol content of what you were drinking? Are you developing an allergy to sulfites in wine? Did you set out with the intention of getting sloshed? Sometimes, even though you're used to two glasses, the circumstances might be such that those two glasses cause a headache the next day. Don't rule out the possibility that you overindulged.

Make sure you're eating right and also that you are moving your bowels. Constipation is an issue that can definitely contribute to headaches. We should be having 1-3 bowel movements <u>every day</u>. If you are having fewer or needing to strain, look into a cleanse, colonic, or change in diet. Also, if you are constipated AND get headaches, you might be deficient in magnesium. This important nutrient relaxes smooth muscle and may alleviate both problems. Blood sugar drops and being dehydrated can also lead to headaches. Keep your nutrition balanced and of high quality.

What if your headaches continue or get more frequent or severe? Seek out medical help, as the headaches could be caused by something serious like meningitis, vision problems, MS, a tumor, or cancer. Usually headaches are innocent, but in some cases, they might be a symptom of a more serious problem. Sudden, severe headache or sudden headache associated with a stiff neck; headaches associated with fever, convulsions, or accompanied by confusion or loss of consciousness; headaches following a blow to the head, or associated with pain in the eye or ear; persistent headache in a person who was previously headache free; and recurring headache in children indicate that you should seek medical attention.

Now, what can we do if we find ourselves plagued by the occasion pain in the noggin? Since stress is a common cause, do what you can to decrease it in your life. Meditation, taking time for you, and spending time with friends can lead to less stress and a lessening of headaches. Muscle tension goes hand in hand with stress, so try getting a massage to relax those tight neck, shoulder, and jaw muscles. Many massage therapists like myself have helped their clients eliminate headaches. As mentioned above, think about seeing a chiropractor to help with any alignment issues you might be experiencing. An acupuncturist can do some needling to relieve stress and balance the subtle energy in the body that might be causing the headaches. Often, these types of practitioners can also recommend stretches to help relieve the muscle tension that may be contributing to your headache. And especially if you work at a desk all day, make sure you take time out to stretch and never hold the phone against your ear while you do other things—this is a sure-fire way to throw your neck out of place and create extra muscle tension.

Your Chinese medicine practitioner might also recommend some Chinese herbs to help deal with your symptoms. American herbs can help too. Taking feverfew on a daily basis has been shown to decrease headaches. Some people also recommend sniffing fresh lavender at the first hint of a headache. A homeopathic practitioner also might have some options for you, or a combination remedy can be purchased in most health food stores that contain the most common headache remedies. If you are going to consult with a homeopath, make sure to keep track of the specifics of your headache: what seems to aggravate it, time of day, what relieves it, do you crave certain foods or situations, and any other details you can note. These will help the practitioner hit on the right remedy for your specific headache.

I hope this helps you deal with your headaches and gives you some ideas and solutions.

Repetitive Stress Injuries

We are hearing more and more about repetitive stress injuries (RSIs). If you are a worker in the US, you have a 1 in 8 chance of getting a repetitive stress injury, and they make up the largest single category of workplace injuries. Now, it's not just carpal tunnel and tennis elbow—we have everything from BlackBerry thumb to gamer's thumb. As we get more and more sophisticated with our gadgets and they become smaller and smaller, I think we're going to see more and more of these types of injuries.

Symptoms of RSIs include numbness, tingling or burning sensations, weakness, inability to grip, shooting pains, and increased pain at night. This can occur in the fingers, hands, or forearms and can become crippling. Victims of full-blown RSI cannot wash their hair or even hold a sheet of paper without agonizing pain.

My first recommendation for dealing with the symptoms is to limit the activity causing the problem. Stretch, vary your activities and, if your issue is occurring at work, don't do a similar activity at home. Give your hands a break. I had a client who typed about 10 hours a day. Her leisure activities at home were gardening, knitting, and playing the flute. Way too much hand activity.

Ice is useful for the inflammation and swelling, and alternating ice and heat can bring healing blood to the area. Don't apply heat if there is swelling or you feel heat emanating from the joint. Some creams, like ones with arnica and comfrey, can help.

Seek out alternative therapies like acupuncture, massage, and chiropractic to keep the body properly aligned. Some people find it useful to wear a splint or ace bandage during activities.

Something you might not have thought about is how you sleep. Many people curl their wrists under them in bed. Try to be aware of your positioning and don't sleep on your arms. Wearing a splint or brace for a few nights can sometimes break you of that habit.

Western medicine can offer cortisone shots, surgery, and anti-inflammatory drugs. Sometimes surgery is the answer, but in the case of carpal tunnel syndrome, often the scar tissue that forms following surgery fills in the area that the surgeon just cleaned out. If you do choose to go with surgery, do the recommended physical therapy, seek out massage on your own, and make sure you correct the environmental problems. If you have the surgery and then go right back to the same bad posture and incorrect work station, you're just guaranteed future problems.

Supplementing with vitamin B6 and omega-3 fatty acids has been shown to assist with the symptoms of repetitive stress disorders. Maintaining a healthy weight and keeping up on your exercise is also a necessity. I've read articles talking about the benefits of yoga on RSIs. The only caution I give with that particular type of exercise is be careful putting too much weight on the wrists. Holding the positions down dog and up dog can irritate already overworked wrists and elbows.

It wouldn't be written by me without mentioning the mind/body connection. Do you feel like your hands are full? Can't get a grip? Is there something you need to let go? Or loosen your grip on? Are you grasping at straws? Feel like something is slipping through your fingers or is just out of your grasp? Phrases like this, that we've agreed upon in this society, can be very telling about your physical condition. It's not just enough to address our dis-eases from a physical perspective. We have to look at the emotional components also. Dealing with our conditions from a holistic perspective of body, mind, and spirit will help ensure full and complete healing.

And here are some workplace suggestions specifically to help deal with RSI:
- Use a softer touch on the keys, don't bang them.
- Make sure the desk is set up for good sightline at the monitor or project you are working on and that the chair is adjusted for your height and body mechanics.
- Keep your shoulders relaxed and down when using the keyboard and mouse. Don't hike them up to your ears.
- For any type of job, take at least one break per hour.
- If you are using power tools, make sure they have soft grips and something to absorb the shock, if possible.

- Vary your activities so you don't do the same action all day.
- Get help the second you feel something coming on. Don't wait until it's full blown.
- If you are feeling pain, numbness, tingling, burning, weakness...these are signs something may be wrong. Have it checked out. This is not the time to power through.

Mind/Body Medicine for Pain Management

We have all felt pain, whether we hit our thumb with a hammer or woke up with a headache. I know this is a book about workplace issues, but I wanted to include a section on mind-body therapies for pain management as my background is in massage and helping people deal with their pain. And pain is definitely going to inhibit our ability to do our job.

Pain is usually a signal that something is wrong. But some people find themselves having a chronic pain syndrome. There are also diseases and disorders like fibromyalgia, osteoarthritis, and rheumatoid arthritis that can cause incredible pain in the body. We know that everyone perceives pain differently and everyone has a different pain tolerance or threshold. There are also theories that thoughts and emotions directly influence physiological responses like muscle tension, blood flow, and levels of brain chemistry. It's also suggested that stressful thoughts lead to pain in vulnerable parts of the body, as I mentioned previously.

Anticipation of pain can make it worse. For example, if you start to feel a bad headache coming on, the stress of it hurting or what it's going to do to your day can actually make it worse. Avoiding things that we think may hurt us can also indirectly cause pain by reducing blood flow and muscle tone. The other thing we have to consider is secondary gain. Is there something good you're getting from staying sick?

Here are some specific mind/body techniques for pain. Depending on the type of pain, massage can be incredibly useful. Though in that case you would probably be using it strictly as a physical modality, it does calm and soothe the nervous system as well as smooth out muscle tension and help feel-good hormones in the brain erase that pain response. Massage is good for repetitive stress injuries, back pain, neck and shoulder pain, muscle tension, and stress. Go to a qualified practitioner, not some non-English-speaking shopping center massage parlor, and be very open about what the problem is. Make sure the practitioner understands what you are looking for.

Reiki is also good for pain and can be very good at connecting the mind and body and helping calm the emotions and spirit when chronic pain is present. It also can decrease pain. I had a friend visiting from Los Angeles who had twisted his ankle the day before. We were sitting in a bar with friends having a drink and he was complaining about the pain. I asked him to put his leg up on my mine and I put my hands on his ankle. I sent Reiki for about 15 minutes before he finally said, "Oh my God, what are you doing?!" He almost sounded angry and I thought I had hurt him. "I'm doing Reiki." I said. "Why, is it hurting?" "No, I don't feel it at all, all the pain is gone." He jumped up and started to walk on it. All the pain was gone. And as a reminder, you can do Reiki on yourself; many people I've trained weren't professionals, but people who wanted it for their own personal life. I know Reiki sounds sort of weird. Energy medicine, what the heck is that? But studies support its efficacy, and many hospitals and cancer centers offer it as a treatment. Give it a shot

Meditation is a remarkable way of decreasing pain response. Multiple studies have been done showing that people who go into a meditative state register less pain in their brains. Whether you do full-blown sit on the pillow meditation or just minis a few times a day, it can help stop your pain. I talk at length about meditation and minis in the companion book, *Conquer Your Stress at Work.*

Visualizing your pain is a wonderful way to help it go away. Whether you picture it as a large lump of ice that is melting, or a block of rock that your inner construction worker is chipping away at, or whether you see angels swooping in to carry it away, studies show that this type of visualization can actually decrease your pain level. One study I remember reading showed an AIDS patient visualizing a radio dial with his pain amount on it. He would then incrementally turn the dial so that it got lower and lower. And his pain actually decreased. We have to remember that programming our minds also programs our bodies.

Don't forget about affirmations for pain management also—changing your mind works. Don't say "I'm no longer in pain." Say, "My neck is stable and healthy." And remember to customize your affirmations and visualization to what works for you.

Anything at all that you can do to relax your body will help with your pain. Often, when we are in pain, we tighten up our muscles in response. This just causes a cyclical event of pain, tension, pain, tension. If you can relax your muscles, your pain will decrease. Doing deep breathing, perhaps with some aromatherapy like lavender, can help decrease the pain response in the body. Deep breathing also gets oxygen into the muscles and the brain and can help with the pain. And sometimes just plain distraction can help.

Depending on what's causing your pain, progressive muscle relaxation can be a great tool. This involves systematically relaxing your body starting with your feet and working your way slowly up the body. And gentle movement like tai chi or yoga can be great for stimulating both the body and mind and calming the nervous system. And don't forget PT.

There are so many non-allopathic ways to help pain; I've mentioned just some of them here. Please explore what works for you and don't feel trapped in a Western Medicine Model or feel like you have to suffer. You can take control and help yourself!

Back Pain

In my practice, the biggest complaint I hear from clients is, "My back hurts." When I ask them if they stretch, they typically answer "No," or, "Not enough." And most admit to sitting too much, either at their office or in the car, so I figure this can apply to a lot of you. Here are some back-care hints.

Give Yourself a Break
It is essential to change position and tasks and move your body throughout the day. We are not made to sit in one posture for very long. It's recommended that you take a break at least every 50 minutes. This might be a quick walk around the block or your office, or simply a three- to five-minute stretch. Do what feels good and don't push yourself to contort your body into positions that are painful. Basic moves like touching your toes, bending from side to side, and stretching out your arms and neck are appropriate. Please see illustrations of stretches earlier in the book.

Chairs
You don't have to own the most expensive chair in the world, but you do have to make sure it fits YOUR body. We are all biologically individual, and what feels good to me might not feel good to you. If you have the option, pick out your own office chair after trying several options in the store. One that has adjustable arms, lumbar support, and variable seat height is ideal. If you can't get a new chair, try to adapt the one you have with pillows or lumbar supports. The same applies to your car seat: take advantage of the built-in adjustments available in your particular car and add additional pillows or lifts as needed to reach maximum comfort and support.

A note about standing desks. Those can be great, but they have their own set of problems. Make sure you have a way to rest your arm on the desk to use the mouse. Don't strain your eyes. And I recommend having a small box that you can put one leg up on and alternate. Usually we stand on our short leg and thrust the long leg out next to us. This can irritate back issues.

Putting one leg up on a small lift can help take pressure off the low back.

No Pain, No Gain

What if even the shortest amount of sitting is a problem for you? It might be that you have a leg-length difference. To some degree, we all have a shorter leg and it doesn't usually bother us. But some really feel it and it causes pain with prolonged standing or sitting. A chiropractor or massage therapist can usually tell you if your pelvis is tilted or legs are uneven. If this turns out to be true for you, using a lift in one shoe or a butt-lift when you are sitting can provide a huge relief. Chiropractors can often correct the leg length difference through treatment.

To determine which is your shorter leg, stand in bare feet and take a small book or magazine about ½ inch thick. Put it under one foot; stand evenly on both feet and see how you feel. Does it make you feel really crooked or even you out? Try it under the other foot. Inevitably, it feels good under one and horrible under the other. (Usually the short leg is the painful side of the back, but not always.) Now that you have determined your short side, use an insole in that one shoe or fold a pillow case and put it under that one side of your bottom when you are sitting. It can make all the difference in the world!

Get Bodywork

Sometimes your back pain might be simply caused by muscle tension or a vertebra that has subluxed, or gone out of alignment. A therapeutic massage can ease the muscle tension and a chiropractor can fix the subluxed vertebrae. You may have been told that you have a herniated disc, ruptured disc, narrowing of the nerve passage, or some other structural problem. I still encourage trying massage with someone who is skilled in handling those types of problems. If the low back is an issue for you, have them put a pillow under your hips when you are lying face down to take the pressure off the low back. And if it hurts...stop! Even though you could potentially have one of those serious structural issues, in some cases it is just the soft tissue that is causing the pain.

I always consider surgery a final resort after trying less invasive modalities. For example, I have had clients diagnosed with herniated discs who were on the verge of undergoing surgery. But after a few massages, the muscles loosened and the pain went away.

Adjustments.
Chiropractic is obviously good for structural issues such as whiplash and sciatica. But Dr. John Craviotto, with over 25 years chiropractic experience, reminds us that other disorders can be helped through adjustments. "Keeping the spine aligned keeps the nervous system functioning at 100%. That helps our immune system and assists us in fighting disease."

Feel like chiropractic is a scam? Dr Craviotto responds, "A racket is when the same treatment plan is prescribed for everyone regardless of what they need. Some people with chronic problems do need to be seen for six months; other people only need to be seen once or twice. The main issue is, is there improvement? You have to trust your chiropractor, just as you do your doctor and your mechanic. If you don't...find someone else."

Men, Low Back or Hip Pain?
Many men come to my office with these complaints, and as they turn to go into the treatment room I see a large protrusion on one butt cheek. It's not a tumor, it's a wallet! And when you sit on it consistently, it can throw your whole body out of alignment. We are designed to be symmetrical and our body will compensate to make that happen. So keep your wallet elsewhere! Women, beware of a heavy purse. It can pull your shoulders out of alignment and cause upper back and neck pain.

Stop Needling Me
Try acupuncture. More and more people are turning to acupuncture for low back pain. Jennifer Henry, RN, LAc, MSN, MAOM (www.theacupuncturelady.com), who suffered from back pain herself, specializes in orthopedic acupuncture and has this to say about needling and back pain: "Acupuncture treats pain by increasing blood and energy flow in the affected tissues while

also stimulating the release of endorphins and other pain-killing neurotransmitters. It has been shown that over time, chronic pain makes changes in the brain's chemistry that reinforces the pain cycle. Acupuncture can relieve pain, reduce or eliminate the need for pain medications, and increase the ability to cope with pain."

Mind/Body Connection
When we think of back pain, we assume that it is a physical problem: we sit too much, we lifted incorrectly, or we overdid that weekend soccer game. I have repeatedly observed a significant connection between the emotions and back pain. Back pain is associated with lack of emotional support, guilt, fear of money and financial support. I was taught that the low back corresponds with issues of sex, money, and personal relationship. Many clients that I see are having major problems in one or more of these areas.

We have a vast vocabulary that supports the idea that the mind and body are connected. For example, we might feel "unsupported," "stabbed in the back," that the "weight of the world is on our shoulders," or that we are "spineless" or "unstable." I believe that sometimes we have pain in our bodies to bring these emotions to the surface so they can be addressed. Or, pain erupts to draw our attention away from uncomfortable emotions like anger and depression. If you have back pain, explore issues of irritation and frustration. Acknowledge your emotions, talk them out, and see if your pain starts to subside.

The Afternoon Slump

We've all observed children playing. We watch for a second and then say, "Gee, I wish I had their energy." And then everyone laughs as they remember what it was like to not tire as quickly as we do now. I am not guaranteeing you'll be running around the playground by morning, but I do have some suggestions that can help boost your energy.

Proper nutrition is key to energy levels. Since most of the food we eat is either processed, irradiated, minerally depleted, genetically modified, sprayed with a chemical, or artificial, I recommend taking a high-quality vitamin and mineral supplement. The B vitamins are essential for good energy. Increasing B6 and B12 is my first suggestion for weary clients. Don't take them too late in the day though, or they may disrupt your sleep.

Getting a wide variety of minerals is also essential. Everyone stresses the importance of calcium, but there are so many more minerals we need, like iron, magnesium, molybdenum, copper, zinc, etc. Taking a good multimineral supplement can help. Also remember that we need protein for energy. Amino acids, which are the building blocks of protein, can be taken in supplement form. I especially recommend this for vegetarians or non-red-meat eaters.

When we hit that afternoon slump, most people reach for the soda or candy bar. We use glucose as an energy source, so often we crave something sweet. Make sure that what you're eating contains real sugar and not high-fructose corn syrup or some artificial sweetener. These trick our bodies into thinking we are getting sugar, but it's really an unusable substance. Whole food snacks like fruits, dates, and juices contain natural sugars. Don't overdo it on the sugar though, or you will crash later and feel worse. And often, what we really need is protein, not sugar, so try a heartier snack.

Ginseng is a natural stimulant that can be taken in herbal form or can be found in specialty beverages. Make sure what you are drinking actually has ginseng and not just a high amount of caffeine. Too much ginseng, like caffeine, can cause a racing heart, palpitations, or nervousness. Again, moderation is the key. And speaking of caffeine, I personally don't believe caffeine is bad if consumed in moderation. Though remember, drowsiness is not a caffeine deficiency! Too much can cause sleep disturbances, jitteriness, heart issues, anxiety, and is often addictive. Ever have that day where you can't get your morning java? How long before that headache kicks in? Try not to have caffeine too late in the day, as it might interrupt your sleep. Or, if you're prone to heart issues or anxiety, consider eliminating it all together.

The newest boosting craze is energy drinks like Red Bull, No Fear™, Full Throttle, and Rockstar. These drinks are high in sugar and caffeine and can lead to a later crash and physical addiction. This is much worse for children than adults. High amounts of caffeine cause extra excretion of calcium, which in young girls can lead to adult onset of osteoporosis.

Another new trend is mixing these energy drinks with alcohol. From a health standpoint, this is a dangerous combination. Alcohol is a depressant and caffeine and sugar are stimulants. Yes, it allows you to drink more alcohol, but this combination could be disastrous as it clouds your judgment as to how drunk you actually are. This can lead to driving with someone intoxicated, taking sexual risks, and increased injury.

I know the last thing you want to do when you are already tired is exercise, but studies consistently show that exercise can actually boost your energy levels. In fact, a recent review of twelve large-scale studies on the connection between exercise and fatigue concluded that all studies found a direct link between physical activity and reduced fatigue for participants who were physically active compared to those who were inactive. Other research shows that even among people with chronic illness like cancer or heart disease, exercise can ward off feelings of fatigue and help people feel more energized. This doesn't mean you have to run five miles. Even 15-20 minutes of walking or light exercise can make a difference.

Since our bodies are 80% water, it is important to keep yourself hydrated. If we wait until we feel the sensation of thirst, it is too late; we're already dehydrated. Drink water throughout the day, which helps with blood flow and removal of toxins. Remember, caffeine is a diuretic, which causes increased output of urine, so caffeinated drinks don't count. Pure water is the best!

We can also boost energy by deep breathing. Oxygen carries energy to our cells, which will give us a natural perk. Try four slow deep breaths (use your abdomen not just your chest) and get a natural high.

It stands to reason that if you are not sleeping well, you are going to have low energy the next day. It's a myth that we need eight hours of sleep. We need as much as we need. Some people are fine on six hours, others need nine or ten. Go to bed when you are tired if at all possible. Don't force yourself to stay awake at night, especially by artificial means. And during the day, if you're really tired and can take a nap, take one. But make it short. Don't sleep too much or you will have trouble sleeping that night. More on sleep in the next chapter.

If we are constantly telling ourselves that we're tired and have no energy, we are just programming the body to behave that way. Change your mind to change your body. Try affirmations like, "I am well-rested and energized," "I am filled with vigor," "My energy is boundless." You will have better results with positive thinking.

If you are finding that your energy is consistently low, make sure there is not an underlying condition like anemia, hypothyroid, adrenal insufficiency, infection, fibromyalgia, low blood sugar, depression, or cancer. Blood tests and a physical exam can help rule out a medical problem. Also check any prescriptions or over-the-counter medications you are taking to see if fatigue might be a side effect.

I hope these ideas help you increase your energy. May your nights be restful and your days filled with boundless energy.

Sleep

Early to bed and early to rise keeps a man healthy, wealthy and wise.

Clearly, Ben Franklin didn't have cats, children, deadlines, a spouse that snored, or a neighbor with a loud dog. Sleep is very important to maintaining good health and keeping us sharp at work. It is during sleep that our bodies regenerate and heal, our minds rest and wander, and through our dreams that our subconscious gets to play. Many ponder how much sleep we really need. There is no right answer to that question. As we grow and age, we need different amounts of sleep, and it is a myth that <u>everyone</u> needs eight hours. Some people function fine on six or seven, while others need nine or ten. And that need tends to change with age and activity level. We are all biologically individual, and the most important things are the quality of our sleep and that we sleep when we are tired. In today's stressful society, more and more people are developing sleep disorders, and there are solutions other than prescription drugs. Here are some tips if you have problems; remember, sleeplessness is not just an Ambien® deficiency.

Daytime activities matter. Limit your caffeine intake and don't use stimulants to force yourself to stay awake, especially at night. We have a very delicate system of biorhythms, and when you start to force yourself to stay awake later than you should, it alters your natural sleep cycle and you may start to experience sleep problems. Energy drinks like RedBull and RockStar only act as a temporary fix. Despite the boost of energy these drinks initially provide, you will eventually crash. They can also be highly addictive.

If you need a boost during the day, try a walk, deep breathing, drinking water, or having a healthy snack like nuts. Often when we hit that afternoon slump, we are dehydrated and just need more water or fresh air. Both transport oxygen in our system, which is needed for energy. Don't reach for sugary snacks, as they too can cause a crash. And avoid long naps, though most people agree that a short one is fine, as long naps can result in evening wakefulness.

Another important component of good sleep is nutrition. Supplements like B vitamins, magnesium, tryptophan, and melatonin may help you sleep. Make sure you don't take B vitamins too late in the day, as they can cause wakefulness. Tryptophan is an essential amino acid that our bodies cannot produce on their own and is one of the hardest to absorb from food sources, especially for vegetarians. It is the precursor to 5HTP, which converts to serotonin, the feel-good hormone in the brain that helps with mood and sleep. Melatonin is another naturally occurring substance that can be taken as a supplement to help with sleep. However, avoid tryptophan or melatonin supplements if you are taking SSRI (Selective Serotonin Reuptake Inhibitor) drugs like Prozac® and follow any dosing instructions on the label.

So, you have cut back on the caffeine, taken tryptophan, and you STILL can't sleep. Let's talk about the sleep environment. Make sure the room is dark and quiet; use a white noise machine or earplugs if the space around you tends to be noisy, and make sure your pillows and mattress are appropriate for your unique body type. The environment is especially important for shift workers.

Try not to do anything exciting before bed, like engaging in strenuous exercise, watching a loud, scary movie, or yelling at the evening news. (Sex is ok.) Instead, choose activities that help you to relax and unwind from your day, like reading a non-work-related book (not on a computer), watching something fun on TV (not the news, which can frustrate us), petting your dog or cat, or taking a bubble bath or soak in the hot tub. It is time to leave the day behind us and rest. I know that can be difficult for those Type-A executives and workaholics, but you have to distract yourself from the day however you can. And avoid excess alcohol at night. Not only is it a depressant, but it can disrupt sleep and cause dehydration.

Our minds seem to be our biggest obstacle to going to sleep. Often when we lay in bed, the dark and quiet gives our mind free reign to run rampant. We dwell on our day, worry about tomorrow, have fatalistic thoughts, wonder if what we did was wrong, question our choices for the future, or simply lie there and do work in our heads. We ponder our to-do list or try to solve that one last problem. We have to find a way to shut off that thinker and relax.

However, this is the toughest barrier to sleep because the mind can be like an unruly child. And there are times we really DO have work to do. What is the solution? As I see it, there are two options: shut up and sleep, or get up and work. I don't think it's bad to get out of bed and deal with things. To lie for hours thinking about something is pointless; get up and finish the paper, write stuff down, make a list for tomorrow, check to see if you actually made the deposit in the bank. These things are just going to drive you nuts if you don't address them, so go do them and then return to bed. Or, just get up and distract yourself: read your book until you're tired, watch TV, do a Sudoku—anything to take your mind off the repeating thoughts. Meditation is another popular method for shutting off the mind. There are tapes available that you can play that lead you through a guided meditation to help relax your mind.

Or, try to change your thought patterns. We can only think one thing at a time. So, if you are thinking about something negative or work-related, change the thought to something else. This is what counting sheep is all about; it distracts the mind from other repetitive thoughts. Positive affirmations are another valuable tool to change thought patterns. If I find something is bothering me, I will change the thought to, "I fall asleep quickly and easily," or "I awake feeling refreshed." These affirmations not only distract you from the problem thoughts, but also program the body. Remember the mind/body connection and that we are the boss of them both.

Lastly, I would like to suggest some herbs and homeopathic remedies. I recommend trying these before turning to the doctor for a prescription. Herbal teas containing hops, lavender, chamomile, and valerian root are great for sleep. There are also some wonderful homeopathic formulas like Moon Drops that allow you to drift off and not wake up feeling groggy. I encourage you to experiment and see what works best for you. Pleasant dreams!

Shift Work

This is a tough one, and I don't offer any quick fixes. Some people are just better at this than others, and it seems that age plays a part in how we handle shift work. Younger folk can do it more easily. My best advice is to try to keep your life as normal as possible. When you get off work, go straight home and straight to bed. Don't go shopping or head off to a meal with the guys. Get in your bed and have great sleep hygiene. A dark room with blackout curtains, quiet or a white noise machine, don't have anyone bother you. They may think they are being quiet when they come in to feed the fish, but you stir more easily if you are on opposite cycles than the rest of the world. Try to avoid stimulants to keep yourself awake, especially near the end of your shift, and stick to the best nutrition possible.

Telecommuting

A new and interesting issue is with people that telecommute or work from home. There are a few special issues with this. Often, the desk set up is subpar or non-existent. Try not to treat your dining room table or slouch on the couch as your office. Get an adjustable desk and a chair that fits your body. Bolster with pillows, blocks, or books to make sure everything is at the perfect height, distance, and level for you.

Another issue with working at home is, you never leave work. It's very tempting to do one of two things. You get distracted with home stuff like, I'll just do one more dish or hey, the cat seems needy. Or you are always working, to the exclusion of "going home." I suggest leaving the house in the morning, walking or driving around, arriving at "work," and then doing the reverse at night. Set as normal hours as you can, depending on your job. And make it known that when you are working, you are not to be bothered. Close the door, hang something on it, etc., to signal that it is work hours for you. And try to find balance with stopping when you have to. The downside of the great convenience of having phones that do everything is there is no reason we can't lay in bed at 2am and respond to email. I sort of miss the good ol' days of M-F, 9-5 and if you missed those hours, you had to wait. Now it's expected to be available almost 24/7 and it's unhealthy and unrealistic. Set the boundaries that you need to, with both your family and your job (or yourself, if you are your own boss).

Work/Life Balance:
How to Leave Work at Work and Home at Home

I just wanted to touch on this subject briefly, as it could fill a whole book on its own. When it comes to balancing work and home, you have to make choices. It's actually pretty simple. You have to choose to put yourself on the list. You have to choose to perhaps stand up to your boss and say, "No, I can't work on Sunday, my kid has a soccer game." You have to choose to say, "Honey, can you watch the kids tonight? I really want to go dance with some friends." I've had clients express that they feel guilty when they take time for themselves. What message is that sending your children? And what is that doing to your health? We choose where we put our focus, what we think about, and what actions we take.

And it's not only important to leave work at work, but also to leave your stresses and negativity about outside issues out of the workplace. Your job is not the place to complain about your spouse, your other job, THIS job, or the kids. Do we have bad days where we have to vent for five minutes? Absolutely, but you can't make it your daily mantra. I advise people to spend 5 minutes in the car between work and home. Tell your spouse/partner/coworker/roommate that you are going to take just five minutes as a transition. Maybe you meditate. Maybe you list things you need to do or are mad at or are grateful for. Maybe you blare NIN (I'm very familiar with this one), but use that as your time to transition.

If you don't drive to work, do this on the bus while wearing headphones, take an extra walk around the block before you get to your destination. Find the time to do what YOU need to do to transition from home to work and vice versa. Look, it comes down to you. It does. No one can make you do any of the things I've suggested. I can't throw out your soda, buy you live plants, follow you around and make you stretch, or buy you a better chair. It's all up to you. Make that choice, right now, to be healthier. At home and at work. And when you're ready to that, you can sign the health contract on the next page.

Health Contract

I, _____, promise to make the best choices I can at home and at work. I promise to stretch, eat better, and take breaks. I acknowledge that it's my choice to make these changes and that no one can do it but me. And because I love and respect myself, I choose to make them.

Signed:

Date:

Witness:

About the Author

Kathy Gruver, PhD is a motivational speaker, an award-winning author, and hosts the national TV show based on her first book, *The Alternative Medicine Cabinet* (Winner Beverly Hills Book Awards). She earned her PhD in Natural Health and has authored seven books, including *Conquer Your Stress at Work*, *Body/Mind Therapies for the Bodyworker*, *Conquer Your Stress with Mind/Body Techniques* (Winner Indie Excellence Awards, Beverly Hills Book Awards, Global E-book Awards, Irwin Awards, Finalist for the USA Best Books Award), *Journey of Healing* (Winner USA Best Book Awards, Beverly Hills Book Awards, Pinnacle Awards, Indie Excellence Awards, and the non-fiction category of the London Book Festival), and she co-wrote *Market My Practice.*

She has studied mind/body medicine at the famed Benson-Henry Institute for Mind-Body Medicine at Harvard Medical School and has been featured as an expert in numerous publications, including *Glamour, Fitness, Time, More, Women, Wall Street Journal, CNN, WebMD, Prevention, Huffington Post, Yahoo.com, Marie Claire, Ladies Home Journal,* Dr. Oz's *The Good Life,* and *First.* Dr. Gruver has appeared as a guest expert on over 250 radio and TV shows, including NPR, SkyNews London, Every Way Woman, Morning Blend in Las Vegas, CBS Radio, and Lifetime Television, and has done over 150 educational lectures around the world for everyone from nurses in the Middle East to 911 dispatchers in New Orleans, corporations around the US, and teachers in her own backyard. She was thrilled to appear on the TEDx stage. Recently, she was honored to work on a project for the military to create and institute a stress-reduction program. For fun and stress relief, Dr. Gruver does flying trapeze and hip-hop dance.

Dr. Gruver maintains a massage and hypnotherapy practice in Santa Barbara, California. She has also produced an instructional massage DVD, *Therapeutic Massage at Home: Learn to Rub People the RIGHT Way™,* and is a practitioner with over 25 years of experience. More information can be found at www.KathyGruver.com

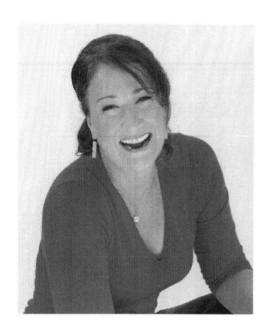

Made in the USA
Middletown, DE
02 May 2022

65073001R00040